THE INVISIBLE ENEMY

A Medical and Historical Perspective on

Bacterial Infections

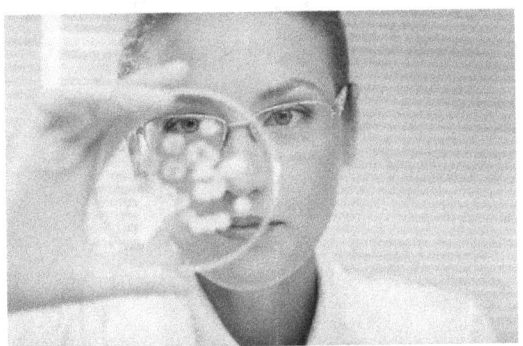

Tim A. Nakashima

Copyright © 2023 Tim A. Nakashima, All Rights Reserved

No part of this publication may be reproduced, distributed, or transmitted in any form or by any means, including photocopying, recording, or other electronic or mechanical methods, without the prior written permission of the publisher.

All trademarks, copyrights, and other intellectual property belong to their respective owners. All rights reserved.

TABLE OF CONTENT

- Introduction

- Chapter 1

The History of Bacterial Infections

- Chapter 2

The Role of Bacteria in Human Health and Disease

II. Types of Bacterial Infections

- Chapter 3

Gastrointestinal Infections

- Chapter 4

Skin and Soft Tissue Infections

- Chapter 5

Genitourinary Infections

- Chapter 6

Respiratory Infections

- Chapter 7

Other Types of Bacterial Infections

III. Diagnosis and Treatment of Bacterial Infections

- Chapter 8

Viral Infection

- Chapter 9

Fungal infection

- Chapter 10

Alternative and Complementary Treatments for Bacterial Infections

IV. Prevention and Control of Bacterial Infections

- Chapter 11

The History of Infectious Diseases

- Chapter 12

The Future of Infectious Diseases

- Chapter 13

Key Takeaways and Recommendations for the Public

- Conclusion

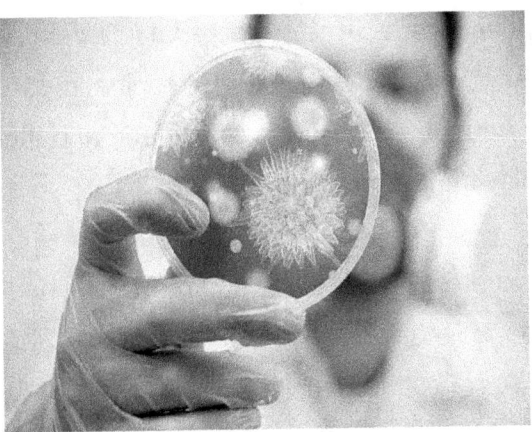

INTRODUCTION

Welcome to "The Invisible Enemy: A Medical and Historical Perspective on Bacterial Infections"! In this book, we will delve into the fascinating and often misunderstood world of bacteria and the role they play in human health and disease.

Bacteria are all around us, and they have been a part of the Earth's ecosystem for billions of years. While some bacteria are beneficial and even essential to human life, others can cause serious infections that can lead to illness and even death. Bacterial infections have plagued humanity for centuries, and they continue to pose a significant threat to public health today.

In this book, we will explore the history of bacterial infections and how they have affected societies around the world. We will also examine the different types of bacterial infections and how they are diagnosed and treated. Additionally, we will discuss the importance of prevention and control measures in reducing the incidence of bacterial infections.

So let's dive in and learn more about these microscopic organisms and the important role they play in our lives.

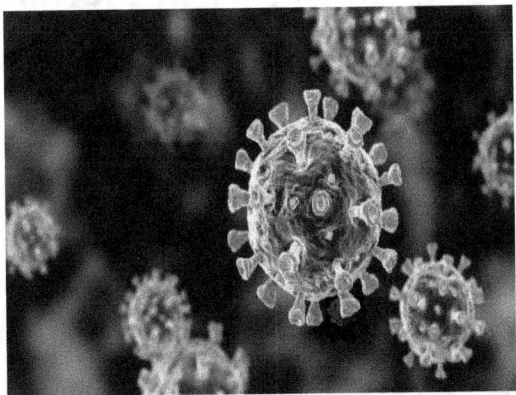

CHAPTER 1

The History of Bacterial Infections

Bacteria have been a part of the Earth's ecosystem for billions of years, and they have played a significant role in the evolution and development of life on our planet. However, it was not until the late 19th century that bacteria were discovered and identified as the cause of many infectious diseases.

The history of bacterial infections is a long and fascinating one, and it is intertwined with the history of medicine and public health. Throughout the centuries, bacterial infections have caused widespread epidemics and pandemics that have had a profound impact on human society.

One of the earliest recorded outbreaks of a bacterial infection occurred in 430 BCE, during the Peloponnesian War between Athens and Sparta. A deadly disease known as the "Plague of Athens" swept through the city, killing an estimated 75,000 people. It is believed that the disease was caused by the bacterium Yersinia pestis, which is the same bacterium that causes the plague today.

Another major outbreak of a bacterial infection occurred in the 14th century, when the "Black Death" or bubonic plague swept through Europe, killing millions of people. The plague was caused by Yersinia pestis and was transmitted to humans through the bite of infected fleas that lived on rats.

In the 19th and 20th centuries, several major bacterial infections emerged, including cholera, typhoid fever, and tuberculosis. These diseases caused widespread epidemics and claimed the lives of millions of people. However, the development of vaccines and antibiotics in the 20th century greatly reduced the incidence of these diseases and greatly improved public health.

Despite these advances, bacterial infections continue to be a major public health threat. In recent years, new strains of bacteria have emerged that are resistant to antibiotics, and outbreaks of bacterial infections continue to occur. It is important for us to continue to educate ourselves about these diseases and take steps to prevent and control them.

In the modern era, bacterial infections remain a significant public health threat, and they can have a major impact on communities and societies around the world. In the 21st century, several major outbreaks of bacterial infections have occurred, including the 2002-2004 SARS outbreak, the 2009 H1N1 influenza pandemic, and the ongoing COVID-19 pandemic.

SARS, or severe acute respiratory syndrome, was caused by a virus called the SARS coronavirus, which is a type of virus that belongs to the same family as the coronavirus that causes COVID-19.

The SARS outbreak originated in China and spread to other countries, causing over 8,000 confirmed cases and 774 deaths.

The H1N1 influenza pandemic, also known as the "swine flu," was caused by a strain of influenza virus that was first detected in Mexico and the United States in 2009. The virus spread rapidly around the world, and it is estimated that it infected over 1 billion people and caused hundreds of thousands of deaths.

The COVID-19 pandemic, which began in late 2019, is caused by the SARS-CoV-2 virus, which is a member of the coronavirus family. The virus has spread to almost every country in the world and has infected millions of people, resulting in hundreds of thousands of deaths.

Bacterial infections can have a major impact on individuals and communities, and it is important for us to be aware of these diseases and take steps to prevent and control them. This includes practicing good hygiene, getting vaccinated, and following public health guidelines. By understanding the history and current state of bacterial infections, we can work together to protect ourselves and others from these diseases.

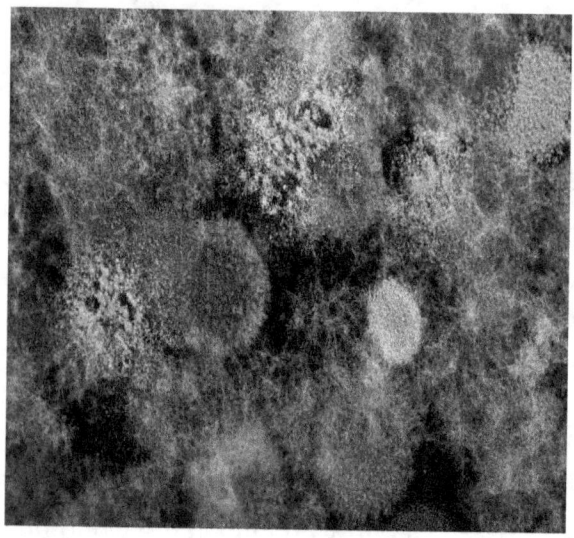

CHAPTER 2

The Role of Bacteria in Human Health and Disease

Bacteria are tiny, single-celled organisms that can be found almost everywhere on Earth. They play a vital role in the ecosystem and have a profound impact on human health and disease. While some bacteria are beneficial and even essential to human life, others can cause serious infections that can lead to illness and even death.

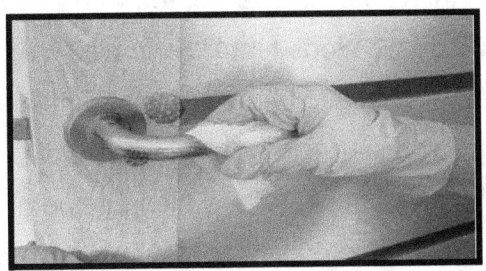

The human body is home to a diverse community of bacteria, known as the microbiome. These bacteria live in various parts of the body, including the skin, mouth, gut, and respiratory tract. The microbiome is a complex and dynamic ecosystem that plays a critical role in human health and well-being.

On the other hand, harmful bacteria, also known as pathogens, can cause infections and other health problems. Pathogenic bacteria can enter the body through various routes, such as the mouth, respiratory tract, or skin. Once inside the body, they can multiply and cause damage to tissues and organs. Bacterial infections can range from mild to severe and can affect different parts of the body.

Bacterial infections can be treated with antibiotics, which are medications that kill or inhibit the growth of bacteria. However, the overuse and misuse of antibiotics can lead to the development of antibiotic-resistant bacteria, which can be difficult to treat. It is important to use antibiotics responsibly and only when they are needed to help reduce the risk of antibiotic resistance.

In conclusion, bacteria play a complex and multifaceted role in human health and disease. While some bacteria are beneficial and essential to human life, others can cause serious infections. It is important to understand the role of bacteria in health and disease and to take steps to prevent and control bacterial infections.

In addition to their role in human health and disease, bacteria also play a vital role in the ecosystem. They are involved in many important ecological processes, such as decomposition, nitrogen fixation, and the cycling of nutrients. Without bacteria, many of these processes would not occur, and the ecosystem would not function properly.

Bacteria are also important in many industrial and technological applications. They are used in the production of a variety of products, such as food, beverages, and pharmaceuticals. They are also used in environmental remediation, bioremediation, and biotechnology.

Despite their importance, bacteria can also be a source of concern and fear for many people. This is often due to the negative connotations associated with bacteria and the diseases they can cause. However, it is important to remember that not all bacteria are harmful, and many of them play a vital role in human health and the ecosystem.

In summary, bacteria are a diverse and ubiquitous group of organisms that play a vital role in human health and disease, as well as in the ecosystem. They are involved in many important ecological processes and have a wide range of industrial and technological applications. Understanding the role of bacteria in health and disease can help us to better prevent and control bacterial infections and to appreciate the vital role that these organisms play in our lives.

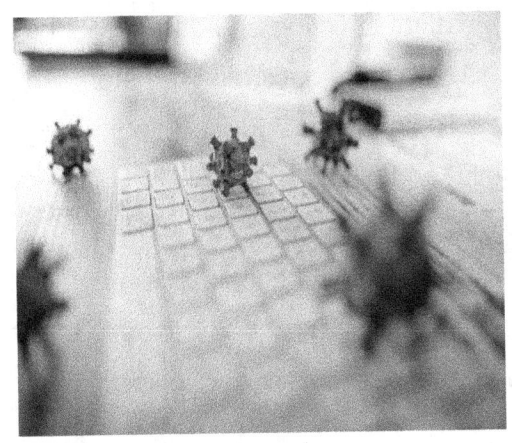

Types of bacterial infection

There are many different types of bacterial infections, and they can affect different parts of the body. Some common types of bacterial infections include:

Respiratory infections: These infections affect the respiratory system, including the lungs, throat, and sinuses. Examples include pneumonia, bronchitis, and sinusitis.

Gastrointestinal infections: These infections affect the digestive system, including the stomach and intestines. Examples include food poisoning, salmonella, and E. coli.

Skin and soft tissue infections: These infections affect the skin and the tissues beneath it. Examples include impetigo, cellulitis, and folliculitis.

Genitourinary infections: These infections affect the reproductive and urinary systems. Examples include urinary tract infections, sexually transmitted infections, and prostatitis.

Central nervous system infections: These infections affect the brain and spinal cord. Examples include meningitis and encephalitis.

Other types of bacterial infections: There are many other types of bacterial infections that can affect different parts of the body, including bone infections, blood infections, and eye infections.

Bacterial infections can range from mild to severe, and they can be treated with antibiotics. It is important to see a healthcare provider if you suspect that you have a bacterial infection and to follow their recommended treatment plan.

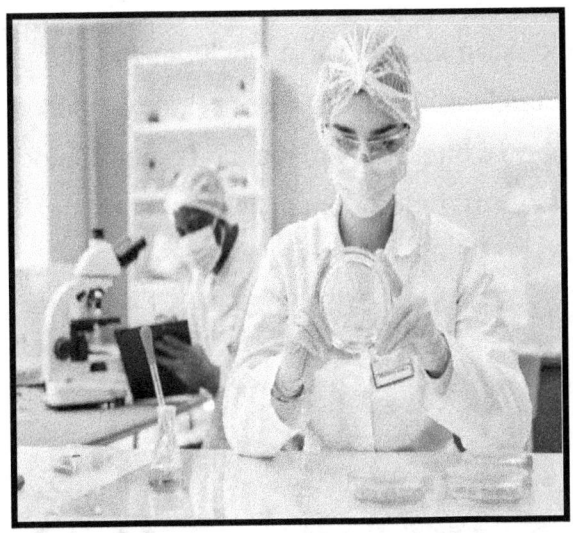

CHAPTER 3

Gastrointestinal Infections

Gastrointestinal infections are infections that affect the digestive system, which includes the stomach and intestines. These infections can be caused by a variety of bacteria, viruses, and other pathogens, and they can range from mild to severe.

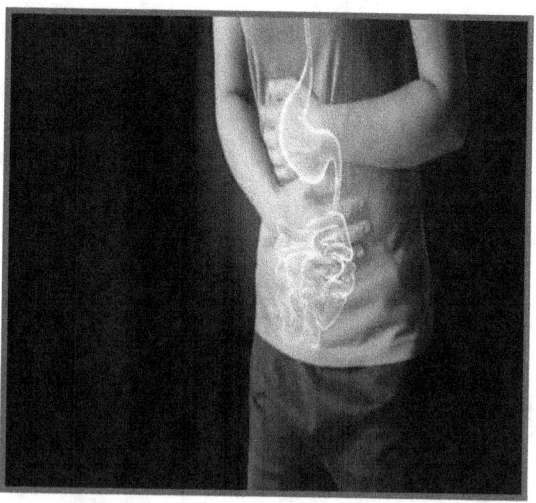

Some common types of gastrointestinal infections include:

Food poisoning: Food poisoning is an illness caused by eating food that is contaminated with bacteria, viruses, or other toxins. Symptoms of food poisoning include nausea, vomiting, diarrhea, and abdominal cramps. Food poisoning can be treated with over-the-counter medications and home remedies, but it can sometimes be serious, especially for older adults, young children, and people with weakened immune systems.

Salmonella: Salmonella is a bacterial infection that affects the digestive system. It is often transmitted through contaminated food, such as undercooked meat, eggs, or produce. Symptoms of salmonella include diarrhea, abdominal cramps, fever, and vomiting. Salmonella can be treated with antibiotics, but it can be serious, especially for people with compromised immune systems.

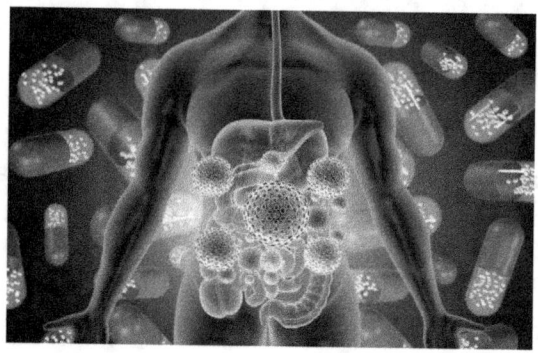

E. coli: E. coli is a type of bacteria that can cause infections of the digestive system. It is often transmitted through contaminated food or water and can cause symptoms such as diarrhea, abdominal cramps, and fever. E. coli infections can range from mild to severe, and they can sometimes lead to serious complications such as kidney failure.

Gastrointestinal infections can be prevented by practicing good hygiene, such as washing your hands frequently and cooking food properly. It is also important to drink clean, safe water and to avoid consuming raw or undercooked food. If you suspect that you have a gastrointestinal infection, it is important to see a healthcare provider for proper diagnosis and treatment.

Other types of gastrointestinal infections include:

Norovirus: Norovirus is a viral infection that affects the digestive system. It is often transmitted through contaminated food or water and can cause symptoms such as diarrhea, vomiting, and abdominal cramps. Norovirus is highly contagious and can spread rapidly through close contact with infected individuals. There is no specific treatment for norovirus, but symptoms can be managed with over-the-counter medications and home remedies.

Helicobacter pylori: Helicobacter pylori is a type of bacteria that can cause infections of the digestive system. It is often transmitted through contaminated food or water and can cause symptoms such as abdominal pain, nausea, and loss of appetite. H. pylori infections can lead to serious complications such as ulcers and stomach cancer. H. pylori infections can be treated with a combination of antibiotics and other medications.

Clostridium difficile: Clostridium difficile (C. diff) is a type of bacteria that can cause infections of the digestive system, particularly in people who have recently taken antibiotics. C. diff infections can cause symptoms such as diarrhea, abdominal pain, and fever. C. diff infections can be serious, especially for older adults and people with weakened immune systems, and they can be difficult to treat.

In summary, gastrointestinal infections are infections that affect the digestive system and can range from mild to severe. They can be caused by a variety of pathogens, including bacteria, viruses, and toxins, and they can be prevented by practicing good hygiene and avoiding contaminated food and water. If you suspect that you have a gastrointestinal infection, it is important to see a healthcare provider for proper diagnosis and treatment.

In addition to the common gastrointestinal infections listed above, there are many other types of infections that can affect the digestive system. Some of these infections are more rare and can be more severe, such as inflammatory bowel disease (IBD) and gastrointestinal bleeding.

Inflammatory bowel disease (IBD) is a group of chronic conditions that cause inflammation in the digestive tract. The two main types of IBD are ulcerative colitis and Crohn's disease. Symptoms of IBD include abdominal pain, diarrhea, weight loss, and fatigue. IBD is a long-term condition that can be difficult to manage, and it is not always clear what causes it. Treatment for IBD may include medications, surgery, and lifestyle changes.

Gastrointestinal bleeding is the loss of blood from the digestive tract, which can be caused by various conditions such as ulcers, hemorrhoids, or inflammatory bowel disease. Symptoms of gastrointestinal bleeding include black or tarry stools, vomiting blood, and abdominal pain. Gastrointestinal bleeding can be serious and may require hospitalization and treatment with medications or surgery.

In conclusion, gastrointestinal infections are infections that affect the digestive system and can range from mild to severe. They can be caused by a variety of pathogens, including bacteria, viruses, and toxins, and they can be prevented by practicing good hygiene and avoiding contaminated food and water. If you suspect that you have a gastrointestinal infection, it is important to see a healthcare provider for proper diagnosis and treatment. There are also other conditions, such as IBD and gastrointestinal bleeding, that can affect the digestive system and may require specialized treatment.

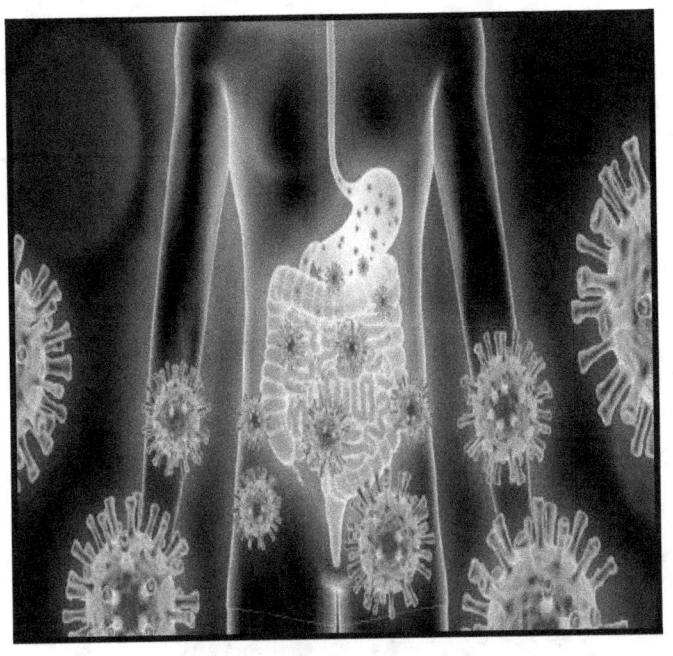

CHAPTER 4

Skin and Soft Tissue Infections

Skin and soft tissue infections are infections that affect the skin and the tissues beneath it. These infections can be caused by a variety of bacteria, viruses, and other pathogens, and they can range from mild to severe.

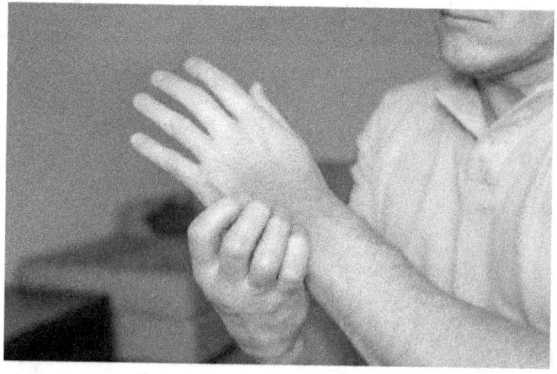

Some common types of skin and soft tissue infections include:

Impetigo: Impetigo is a bacterial infection of the skin that is most common in children. It is characterized by red, itchy sores that contain pus and can spread easily to other parts of the body. Impetigo can be treated with antibiotics, but it is important to keep the sores clean and covered to prevent the infection from spreading.

Cellulitis: Cellulitis is a bacterial infection of the deeper layers of the skin and the underlying tissues. It is characterized by red, swollen, and painful skin that is warm to the touch. Cellulitis can be serious, especially if it spreads to the bloodstream, and it requires prompt treatment with antibiotics.

Folliculitis: Folliculitis is an infection of the hair follicles, which are the small pockets in the skin that contain hair roots. It is characterized by red, itchy bumps on the skin that may contain pus. Folliculitis can be caused by bacteria, fungi, or other pathogens, and it can be treated with antibiotics or antifungal medications.

Skin and soft tissue infections can be prevented by practicing good hygiene, such as washing your hands frequently and keeping cuts and wounds clean and covered. If you suspect that you have a skin or soft tissue infection, it is important to see a healthcare provider for proper diagnosis and treatment.

Other types of skin and soft tissue infections include:

Staphylococcal infections: Staphylococcal infections are infections caused by the bacterium Staphylococcus. They can affect the skin and other parts of the body, such as the respiratory tract, urinary tract, and bloodstream. Staphylococcal infections can range from mild to severe and can be treated with antibiotics.

Herpes infections: Herpes infections are caused by the herpes simplex virus (HSV). They can affect the skin, mucous membranes, and other parts of the body, and they can cause symptoms such as painful blisters, fever, and muscle aches. There is no cure for herpes infections, but they can be managed with antiviral medications.

Fungal infections: Fungal infections are caused by fungi, which are a type of microorganism. They can affect the skin, nails, and other parts of the body, and they can cause symptoms such as itching, redness, and scaling. Fungal infections can be treated with antifungal medications, but they can sometimes be difficult to cure.

In summary, skin and soft tissue infections are infections that affect the skin and the tissues beneath it. They can be caused by a variety of pathogens, including bacteria, viruses, and fungi, and they can range from mild to severe. Skin and soft tissue infections can be prevented by practicing good hygiene, and they can be treated with antibiotics, antiviral medications, or antifungal medications. If you suspect that you have a skin or soft tissue infection, it is important to see a healthcare provider for proper diagnosis and treatment.

In addition to the common skin and soft tissue infections listed above, there are many other types of infections that can affect the skin and underlying tissues. Some of these infections are more rare and can be more severe, such as necrotizing fasciitis and gangrene.

Necrotizing fasciitis is a serious bacterial infection that affects the deeper layers of the skin and the underlying tissues. It is characterized by rapidly spreading tissue death, or necrosis, and it can be life-threatening if not treated promptly. Necrotizing fasciitis is often caused by a type of bacteria called Streptococcus, but it can also be caused by other types of bacteria. Treatment for necrotizing fasciitis may include surgery to remove infected tissue and antibiotics.

Gangrene is a serious condition that occurs when tissue dies due to a lack of blood flow. It can affect the skin and underlying tissues, and it can be caused by infections, injuries, or other conditions that disrupt blood flow. Gangrene can be life-threatening if not treated promptly, and it may require surgery to remove infected tissue.

In conclusion, skin and soft tissue infections are infections that affect the skin and the tissues beneath it. They can be caused by a variety of pathogens, including bacteria, viruses, and fungi, and they can range from mild to severe. Skin and soft tissue infections can be prevented by practicing good hygiene, and they can be treated with antibiotics, antiviral medications, or antifungal medications. If you suspect that you have a skin or soft tissue infection, it is important to see a healthcare provider for proper diagnosis and treatment. There are also other serious conditions, such as necrotizing fasciitis and gangrene, that can affect the skin and underlying tissues and may require specialized treatment.

CHAPTER 5

Genitourinary Infections

Genitourinary infections are infections that affect the reproductive and urinary systems. These infections can be caused by a variety of bacteria, viruses, and other pathogens, and they can range from mild to severe.

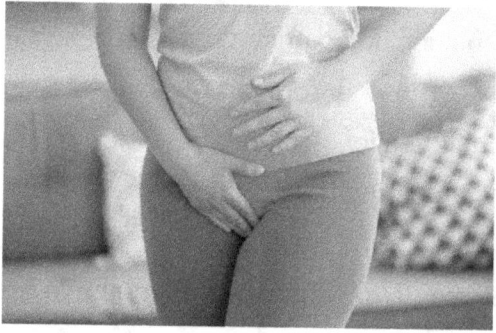

Some common types of genitourinary infections include:

Urinary tract infections: Urinary tract infections (UTIs) are infections of the urinary system, which includes the kidneys, ureters, bladder, and urethra. UTIs are most common in women and are characterized by symptoms such as frequent urination, pain or burning during urination, and abdominal pain. UTIs can be treated with antibiotics, but they can sometimes lead to serious complications such as kidney infection.

Sexually transmitted infections: Sexually transmitted infections (STIs) are infections that are transmitted through sexual contact. They can affect the reproductive and urinary systems, as well as other parts of the body. Examples of STIs include chlamydia, gonorrhea, and syphilis. STIs can be treated with antibiotics, but they can sometimes lead to serious complications such as infertility.

Prostatitis: Prostatitis is an inflammation of the prostate gland, which is a small gland in the male reproductive system. It can be caused by bacteria, viruses, or other pathogens, and it is characterized by symptoms such as pain or discomfort in the pelvic area, difficulty urinating, and fever. Prostatitis can be treated with antibiotics, but it can sometimes be difficult to cure.

Other types of genitourinary infections include:

Vaginal infections: Vaginal infections are infections that affect the vagina, which is the muscular tube in the female reproductive system. They can be caused by bacteria, fungi, or other pathogens, and they are characterized by symptoms such as discharge, itching, and abnormal bleeding. Vaginal infections can be treated with antibiotics or antifungal medications, but they can sometimes lead to serious complications such as infertility.

Pelvic inflammatory disease: Pelvic inflammatory disease (PID) is an infection of the female reproductive organs, including the uterus, fallopian tubes, and ovaries. It is often caused by sexually transmitted infections, such as chlamydia and gonorrhea, and it is characterized by symptoms such as abdominal pain, abnormal bleeding, and fever. PID can be serious, especially if it is not treated promptly, and it can lead to complications such as infertility.

Epididymitis: Epididymitis is an inflammation of the epididymis, which is a small, coiled tube in the male reproductive system. It is often caused by sexually transmitted infections, but it can also be caused by other types of infections or injuries. Epididymitis is characterized by symptoms such as pain or swelling in the testicles, fever, and difficulty urinating. It can be treated with antibiotics, but it can sometimes lead to serious complications such as infertility.

In summary, genitourinary infections are infections that affect the reproductive and urinary systems. They can be caused by a variety of pathogens, including bacteria, viruses, and fungi, and they can range from mild to severe. Genitourinary infections can be prevented by practicing safe sex and good hygiene, and they can be treated with antibiotics, antiviral medications, or antifungal medications. If you suspect that you have a genitourinary infection, it is important to see a healthcare provider for proper diagnosis and treatment. There are also other conditions, such as PID and epididymitis, that can affect the reproductive system and may require specialized treatment.

In addition to the common genitourinary infections listed above, there are many other types of infections that can affect the reproductive and urinary systems. Some of these infections are more rare and can be more severe, such as cystitis and pyelonephritis.

Cystitis is an inflammation of the bladder, which is a muscular sac in the urinary system that stores urine. It is often caused by bacterial infections, but it can also be caused by other types of infections or injuries. Cystitis is characterized by symptoms such as frequent urination, pain or burning during urination, and abdominal pain. It can be treated with antibiotics, but it can sometimes lead to serious complications such as kidney infection.

Pyelonephritis is an infection of the kidneys, which are a pair of organs in the urinary system that filter waste and excess fluids from the blood. It is often caused by bacterial infections, but it can also be caused by other types of infections or injuries. Pyelonephritis is characterized by symptoms such as fever, abdominal pain, and back pain. It can be serious, especially if it is not treated promptly, and it may require hospitalization and treatment with antibiotics.

In conclusion, genitourinary infections are infections that affect the reproductive and urinary systems. They can be caused by a variety of pathogens, including bacteria, viruses, and fungi, and they can range from mild to severe. Genitourinary infections can be prevented by practicing safe sex and good hygiene, and they can be treated with antibiotics, antiviral medications, or antifungal medications. If you suspect that you have a genitourinary infection, it is important to see a healthcare provider for proper diagnosis and treatment. There are also other conditions, such as cystitis and pyelonephritis, that can affect the urinary system and may require specialized treatment.

It is important to note that genitourinary infections can affect both men and women, although some types of infections are more common in one gender than the other. For example, UTIs are more common in women, while prostatitis is more common in men.

In both men and women, genitourinary infections can sometimes lead to serious complications, such as kidney infection, infertility, and sepsis. Kidney infection, also known as pyelonephritis, is an infection of the kidneys that can cause symptoms such as fever, abdominal pain, and back pain. It can be serious, especially if it is not treated promptly, and it may require hospitalization and treatment with antibiotics.

Infertility is the inability to conceive or carry a pregnancy to term. Genitourinary infections, such as STIs and PID, can sometimes cause infertility by damaging the reproductive organs or the fallopian tubes.

Sepsis is a serious and potentially life-threatening condition that occurs when an infection spreads through the bloodstream and causes widespread inflammation in the body. Genitourinary infections, such as UTIs and pyelonephritis, can sometimes lead to sepsis if they are not treated promptly.

In conclusion, genitourinary infections are infections that affect the reproductive and urinary systems. They can be caused by a variety of pathogens, including bacteria, viruses, and fungi, and they can range from mild to severe. Genitourinary infections can be prevented by practicing safe sex and good hygiene, and they can be treated with antibiotics, antiviral medications, or antifungal medications. If you suspect that you have a genitourinary infection, it is important to see a healthcare provider for proper diagnosis and treatment. Genitourinary infections can lead to serious complications, such as kidney infection, infertility, and sepsis, and it is important to seek prompt medical attention to prevent these complications.

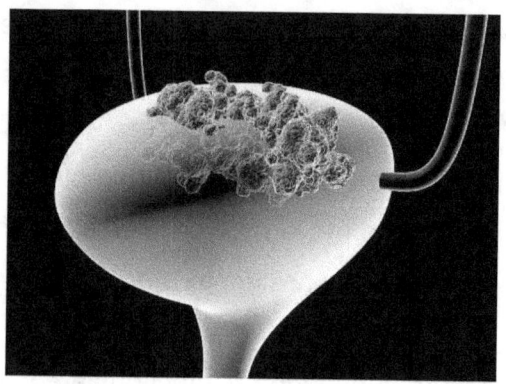

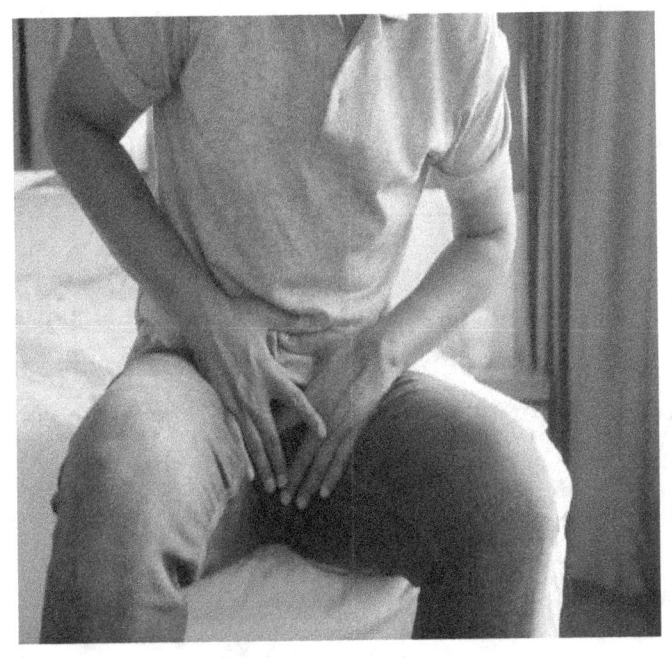

CHAPTER 6

Respiratory Infections

Respiratory infections are infections that affect the respiratory system, which includes the nose, throat, bronchi, and lungs. These infections can be caused by a variety of bacteria, viruses, and other pathogens, and they can range from mild to severe.

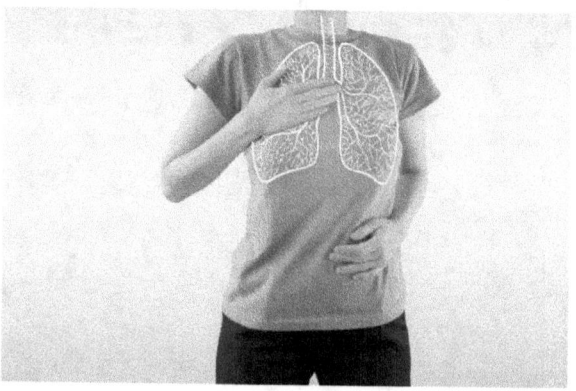

Some common types of respiratory infections include:

Cold: The common cold is a viral infection of the upper respiratory tract, which includes the nose and throat. It is characterized by symptoms such as runny nose, sneezing, and cough. Colds are usually mild and resolve on their own, but they can sometimes lead to more serious infections such as pneumonia.

Influenza: Influenza, also known as the flu, is a viral infection of the respiratory tract. It is characterized by symptoms such as fever, chills, cough, and muscle aches. Influenza can be serious, especially for people with weakened immune systems, and it can lead to complications such as pneumonia. Influenza can be prevented with a vaccine, and it can be treated with antiviral medications.

Pneumonia: Pneumonia is an infection of the lungs that can be caused by bacteria, viruses, or other pathogens. It is characterized by symptoms such as fever, cough, and difficulty breathing. Pneumonia can be serious, especially for people with weakened immune systems, and it may require hospitalization and treatment with antibiotics.

Respiratory infections can be prevented by practicing good hygiene, such as washing your hands frequently and covering your mouth and nose when you cough or sneeze. If you suspect that you have a respiratory infection, it is important to see a healthcare provider for proper diagnosis and treatment.

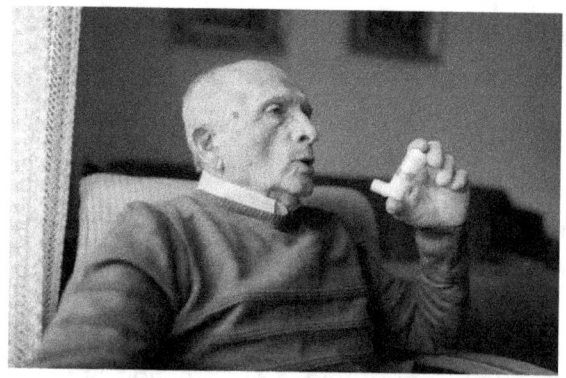

Other types of respiratory infections include:

Bronchitis: Bronchitis is an inflammation of the bronchi, which are the tubes that carry air to and from the lungs. It can be caused by bacteria, viruses, or other pathogens, and it is characterized by symptoms such as cough, phlegm, and difficulty breathing. Bronchitis can be treated with antibiotics, but it can sometimes lead to complications such as pneumonia.

Sinusitis: Sinusitis is an inflammation of the sinuses, which are the small, air-filled cavities in the skull. It can be caused by bacteria, viruses, or other pathogens, and it is characterized by symptoms such as headache, congestion, and nasal discharge. Sinusitis can be treated with antibiotics, but it can sometimes be difficult to cure.

Laryngitis: Laryngitis is an inflammation of the larynx, which is the voice box. It can be caused by bacteria, viruses, or other pathogens, and it is characterized by symptoms such as hoarseness, sore throat, and difficulty speaking. Laryngitis can be treated with antibiotics, but it can sometimes lead to complications such as pneumonia.

In summary, respiratory infections are infections that affect the respiratory system, which includes the nose, throat, bronchi, and lungs. They can be caused by a variety of pathogens, including bacteria, viruses, and fungi, and they can range from mild to severe. Respiratory infections can be prevented by practicing good hygiene, and they can be treated with antibiotics, antiviral medications, or other medications. If you suspect that you have a respiratory infection, it is important to see a healthcare provider for proper diagnosis and treatment. There are also other conditions, such as bronchitis, sinusitis, and laryngitis, that can affect the respiratory system and may require specialized treatment.

In addition to the common respiratory infections listed above, there are many other types of infections that can affect the respiratory system. Some of these infections are more rare and can be more severe, such as tuberculosis and lung abscess.

Tuberculosis (TB) is a bacterial infection that affects the lungs and other parts of the body. It is characterized by symptoms such as fever, night sweats, and weight loss, and it can be serious if not treated promptly. TB is transmitted through the air when an infected person speaks, coughs, or sneezes, and it can be treated with antibiotics.

Lung abscess is a collection of pus in the lung tissue that is caused by a bacterial infection. It is characterized by symptoms such as fever, cough, and difficulty breathing, and it can be serious if not treated promptly. Lung abscess may require hospitalization and treatment with antibiotics, and it may also require surgery to drain the pus.

In conclusion, respiratory infections are infections that affect the respiratory system, which includes the nose, throat, bronchi, and lungs. They can be caused by a variety of pathogens, including bacteria, viruses, and fungi, and they can range from mild to severe. Respiratory infections can be prevented by practicing good hygiene, and they can be treated with antibiotics, antiviral medications, or other medications. If you suspect that you have a respiratory infection, it is important to see a healthcare provider for proper diagnosis and treatment. There are also other conditions, such as TB and lung abscess, that can affect the respiratory system and may require specialized treatment. It is important to seek prompt medical attention for respiratory infections to prevent serious complications.

It is important to note that respiratory infections can affect people of all ages, but they are more common in certain groups of people. For example, respiratory infections are more common in children and in people with weakened immune systems. Children are more likely to get respiratory infections because their immune systems are not fully developed and because they are more likely to be in close contact with other children, who can transmit infections. People with weakened immune systems are more susceptible to respiratory infections because their bodies are less able to fight off infections.

There are several ways to reduce the risk of respiratory infections, including:

Practicing good hygiene: Washing your hands frequently, covering your mouth and nose when you cough or sneeze, and avoiding close contact with sick people can help prevent respiratory infections.

Getting vaccinated: Vaccines can help protect against respiratory infections such as influenza and pneumococcal disease.

Avoiding tobacco smoke: Tobacco smoke can irritate the respiratory system and increase the risk of respiratory infections.

Eating a healthy diet: A healthy diet that is rich in fruits, vegetables, and other nutrients can help support the immune system and reduce the risk of respiratory infections.

Exercising regularly: Regular exercise can help boost the immune system and reduce the risk of respiratory infections.

In conclusion, respiratory infections are infections that affect the respiratory system, which includes the nose, throat, bronchi, and lungs. They can be caused by a variety of pathogens, including bacteria, viruses, and fungi, and they can range from mild to severe. Respiratory infections are more common in certain groups of people, such as children and people with weakened immune systems. There are several ways to reduce the risk of respiratory infections, including practicing good hygiene, getting vaccinated, avoiding tobacco smoke, eating a healthy diet, and exercising regularly. If you suspect that you have a respiratory infection, it is important to see a healthcare provider for proper diagnosis and treatment.

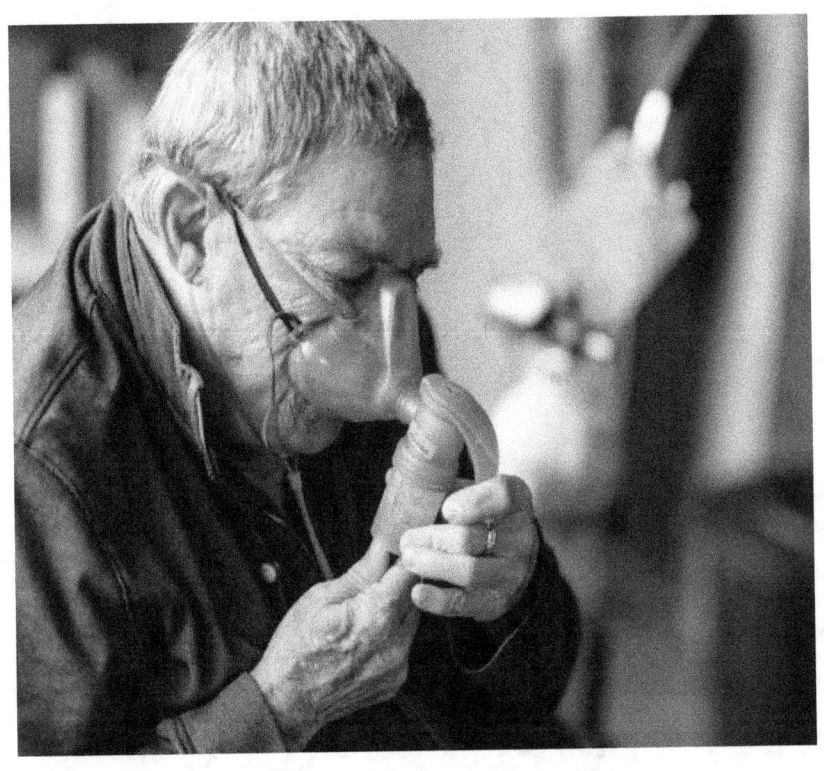

CHAPTER 7

Skin Infections

Skin infections are infections that affect the skin, which is the largest organ in the body. They can be caused by a variety of bacteria, viruses, fungi, and other pathogens, and they can range from mild to severe.

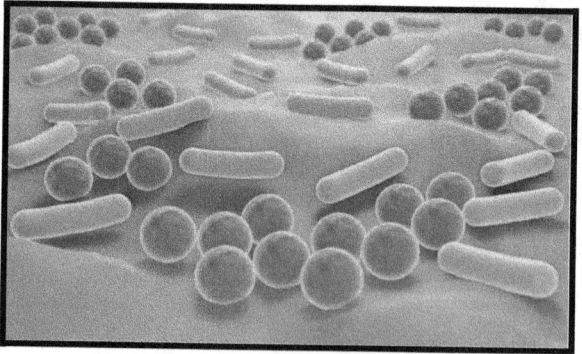

Some common types of skin infections include:

Impetigo: Impetigo is a bacterial infection of the skin that is characterized by red, itchy sores that are filled with pus. It is most common in children and is spread by direct contact with the sores or with objects that have come into contact with the sores. Impetigo can be treated with antibiotics, but it can sometimes lead to more serious infections such as cellulitis.

Cellulitis: Cellulitis is a bacterial infection of the skin and underlying tissues that is characterized by red, swollen, and painful skin. It is usually caused by bacteria that enter the skin through a cut or wound, and it can be serious if not treated promptly. Cellulitis may require hospitalization and treatment with antibiotics.

Folliculitis: Folliculitis is an infection of the hair follicles that is characterized by red, itchy bumps on the skin. It can be caused by bacteria, fungi, or other pathogens, and it can range from mild to severe. Folliculitis can be treated with antibiotics, antifungal medications, or other medications, depending on the cause of the infection.

Skin infections can be prevented by practicing good hygiene, such as washing your hands frequently and keeping cuts and wounds clean. If you suspect that you have a skin infection, it is important to see a healthcare provider for proper diagnosis and treatment.

Other types of skin infections include:

Boils: Boils are infections of the hair follicles that are characterized by red, painful bumps on the skin that are filled with pus. They can be caused by bacteria, such as staphylococcus aureus, and they are most common on the face, neck, armpits, and buttocks. Boils can be treated with antibiotics, but they can sometimes lead to more serious infections such as abscesses.

Abscesses: Abscesses are collections of pus that are caused by infections of the skin or underlying tissues. They are characterized by red, swollen, and painful areas on the skin that are filled with pus, and they can be caused by bacteria, fungi, or other pathogens. Abscesses may require drainage or surgery to remove the pus, and they may also require treatment with antibiotics or other medications.

Herpes: Herpes is a viral infection that is characterized by red, blister-like sores on the skin or mucous membranes. It is caused by the herpes simplex virus and can be transmitted through direct contact with the sores or with bodily fluids such as saliva or genital secretions. Herpes can be treated with antiviral medications, but it cannot be cured.

In summary, skin infections are infections that affect the skin, which is the largest organ in the body. They can be caused by a variety of pathogens, including bacteria, viruses, fungi, and other microorganisms, and they can range from mild to severe. Skin infections can be prevented by practicing good hygiene, and they can be treated with antibiotics, antifungal medications, antiviral medications, or other medications. If you suspect that you have a skin infection, it is important to see a healthcare provider for proper diagnosis and treatment. There are also other conditions, such as boils, abscesses, and herpes, that can affect the skin and may require specialized treatment.

It is important to note that skin infections can affect people of all ages, but they are more common in certain groups of people. For example, skin infections are more common in people with weakened immune systems, in people who have chronic skin conditions such as eczema or dermatitis, and in people who engage in activities that expose them to bacteria or other pathogens, such as gardening or sports.

There are several ways to reduce the risk of skin infections, including:

Practicing good hygiene: Washing your hands frequently and keeping cuts and wounds clean can help prevent skin infections.

Avoiding contact with infected people: Avoiding direct contact with infected people or with objects that have come into contact with infected people can help prevent the spread of skin infections.

Wearing protective clothing: Wearing protective clothing, such as gloves and long sleeves, can help protect the skin from exposure to bacteria and other pathogens.

Using antibiotics appropriately: Using antibiotics only when they are prescribed and needed can help reduce the risk of antibiotic-resistant infections.

Avoiding irritants: Avoiding irritants such as harsh soaps and chemicals can help prevent skin irritation and infections.

In conclusion, skin infections are infections that affect the skin, which is the largest organ in the body. They can be caused by a variety of pathogens, including bacteria, viruses, fungi, and other microorganisms, and they can range from mild to severe. Skin infections are more common in certain groups of people, such as people with weakened immune systems, people with chronic skin conditions, and people who engage in activities that expose them to bacteria or other pathogens. There are several ways to reduce the risk of skin infections, including practicing good hygiene, avoiding contact with infected people, wearing protective clothing, using antibiotics appropriately, and avoiding irritants. If you suspect that you have a skin infection, it is important to see a healthcare provider for proper diagnosis and treatment.

In addition to the common skin infections listed above, there are many other types of infections that can affect the skin. Some of these infections are caused by parasites, such as scabies and lice, and some are caused by fungi, such as athlete's foot and ringworm.

Scabies is a skin infection that is caused by a small mite called Sarcoptes scabiei. It is characterized by a rash of red, itchy bumps on the skin, and it is transmitted through direct contact with infected people or with objects that have come into contact with infected people. Scabies can be treated with medications that kill the mites, such as permethrin, and it can be prevented by avoiding contact with infected people and by washing bedding and clothing in hot water.

Lice are small insects that live on the scalp, body, or pubic area. They are transmitted through direct contact with infected people or with objects that have come into contact with infected people, and they are characterized by itching and the presence of nits (lice eggs) on the hair. Lice can be treated with medications that kill the lice, such as permethrin, and they can be prevented by avoiding contact with infected people and by washing bedding and clothing in hot water.

Athlete's foot is a fungal infection of the skin on the feet that is characterized by red, itchy, and cracked skin. It is caused by a fungus called Trichophyton and is transmitted through contact with infected surfaces or with infected people. Athlete's foot can be treated with antifungal medications, such as terbinafine, and it can be prevented by avoiding contact with infected surfaces and by wearing shoes in public places.

Ringworm is a fungal infection of the skin that is characterized by red, circular, and scaly patches on the skin. It is caused by a fungus called Dermatophytes and is transmitted through contact with infected people or with infected animals. Ringworm can be treated with antifungal medications, such as terbinafine, and it can be prevented by avoiding contact with infected people and animals and by washing bedding and clothing in hot water.

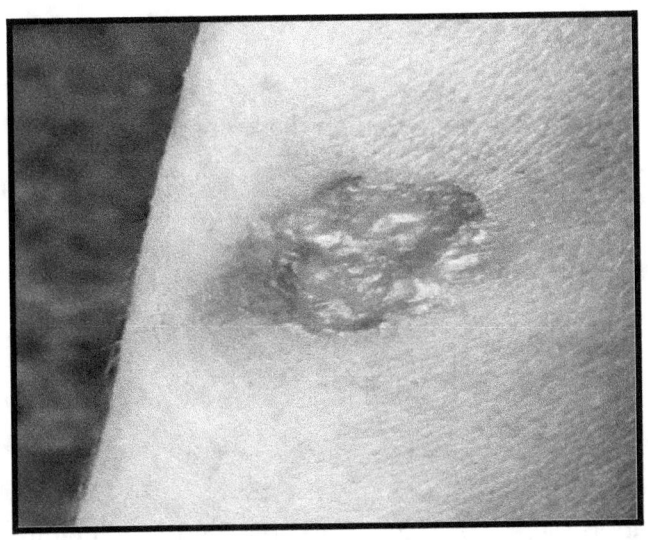

In summary, skin infections are infections that affect the skin, which is the largest organ in the body. They can be caused by a variety of pathogens, including bacteria, viruses, fungi, and other microorganisms, and they can range from mild to severe. There are also other conditions, such as scabies, lice, athlete's foot, and ringworm, that can affect the skin and may require specialized treatment. It is important to practice good hygiene and to avoid contact with infected people and objects to prevent the spread of skin

Diagnosis and Treatment of Bacterial Infections

Bacterial infections can be diagnosed through various methods, including:

Physical examination: A healthcare provider can often diagnose a bacterial infection based on the appearance of the infected area and the presence of specific symptoms.

Laboratory tests: Laboratory tests, such as culture and sensitivity tests, can be used to identify the specific type of bacteria that is causing the infection and to determine the most effective antibiotic to treat the infection.

Imaging tests: Imaging tests, such as X-rays and CT scans, can be used to visualize the infected area and to assess the extent of the infection.

Treatment for bacterial infections typically involves antibiotics, which are medications that kill or inhibit the growth of bacteria. The specific type of antibiotic that is used depends on the type of bacteria that is causing the infection and on the location of the infection. Antibiotics can be administered orally, intravenously, or topically, depending on the severity of the infection and the patient's condition.

It is important to complete the full course of antibiotics as prescribed by a healthcare provider, even if the symptoms of the infection improve. This helps to ensure that all of the bacteria are eliminated and to prevent the development of antibiotic-resistant bacteria.

In conclusion, bacterial infections can be diagnosed through physical examination, laboratory tests, and imaging tests, and they can be treated with antibiotics. It is important to complete the full course of antibiotics as prescribed by a healthcare provider to ensure that all of the bacteria are eliminated and to prevent the development of antibiotic-resistant bacteria. If you suspect that you have a bacterial infection, it is important to see a healthcare provider for proper diagnosis and treatment.

CHAPTER 8

Viral Infections

Viral infections are infections that are caused by viruses, which are tiny infectious particles that can reproduce only inside the living cells of an organism. Viruses can infect all forms of life, including animals, plants, and microorganisms, and they can cause a wide range of diseases.

Some common types of viral infections include:

Influenza: Influenza, or the flu, is a viral infection of the respiratory system that is characterized by fever, cough, sore throat, and body aches. It is caused by the influenza virus and is transmitted through the air when an infected person speaks, coughs, or sneezes, or through contact with infected surfaces. Influenza can be prevented with a vaccine, and it can be treated with antiviral medications such as oseltamivir.

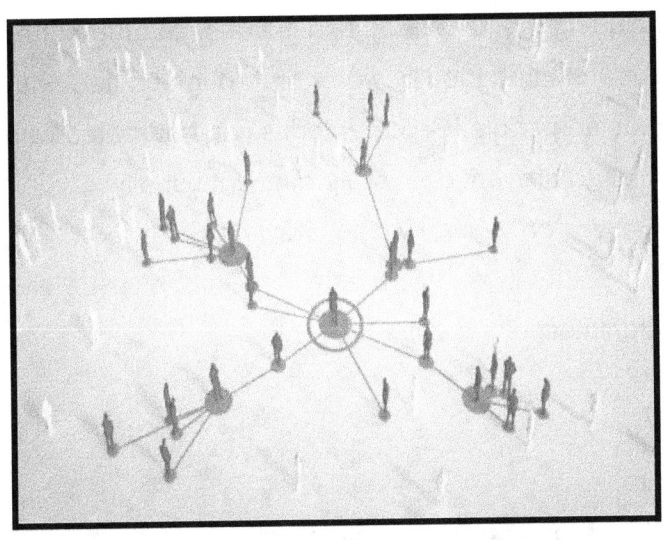

Cold: The common cold is a viral infection of the upper respiratory system that is characterized by symptoms such as runny nose, sneezing, and sore throat. It is caused by a variety of viruses, including the rhinovirus, and is transmitted through the air or through contact with infected surfaces. The common cold has no specific treatment, but it can be relieved with over-the-counter medications such as decongestants and pain relievers.

Gastroenteritis: Gastroenteritis is a viral infection of the gastrointestinal tract that is characterized by symptoms such as diarrhea, vomiting, and abdominal pain. It is caused by a variety of viruses, including the norovirus, and is transmitted through contaminated food or water or through contact with infected people. Gastroenteritis can be treated with fluids to prevent dehydration, and it usually resolves on its own within a few days.

Viral infections can be prevented

Other types of viral infections include:

HIV/AIDS: HIV (human immunodeficiency virus) is a viral infection that attacks the immune system and can lead to AIDS (acquired immune deficiency syndrome). HIV is transmitted through contact with bodily fluids such as blood, semen, vaginal secretions, and breast milk, and it is characterized by symptoms such as fever, rash, and swollen lymph nodes. HIV can be treated with antiviral medications, but it cannot be cured. AIDS is a late stage of HIV infection that is characterized by the development of opportunistic infections and cancers due to the severe suppression of the immune system.

Herpes: Herpes is a viral infection that is characterized by red, blister-like sores on the skin or mucous membranes. It is caused by the herpes simplex virus and can be transmitted through direct contact with the sores or with bodily fluids such as saliva or genital secretions. Herpes can be treated with antiviral medications, but it cannot be cured.

Hepatitis: Hepatitis is a viral infection of the liver that is characterized by symptoms such as jaundice, fatigue, and abdominal pain. It is caused by a variety of viruses, including the hepatitis A, B, and C viruses, and it is transmitted through contaminated food or water or through contact with infected people. Hepatitis can be prevented with vaccines, and it can be treated with antiviral medications or other medications depending on the type of virus.

In summary, viral infections are infections that are caused by viruses, which are tiny infectious particles that can reproduce only inside the living cells of an organism. Viral infections can affect all forms of life and can cause a wide range of diseases. Some common types of viral infections include influenza, the common cold, gastroenteritis, HIV/AIDS, herpes

Viral infections can be more difficult to treat than bacterial infections because viruses are intracellular parasites, which means that they can replicate only inside the cells of an organism. Antibiotics, which are medications that are used to treat bacterial infections, are not effective against viruses because they do not kill viruses or inhibit their replication. Instead, antiviral medications, which are specific to each type of virus, are used to treat viral infections.

There are several ways to reduce the risk of viral infections, including:

Getting vaccinated: Vaccines are designed to stimulate the immune system to produce antibodies that protect against specific viruses. Some vaccines, such as the flu vaccine, are administered annually, while others, such as the hepatitis B vaccine, are administered in a series of doses.

Practicing good hygiene: Washing your hands frequently and avoiding contact with infected people or with objects that have come into contact with infected people can help prevent the spread of viral infections.

Avoiding risky behaviors: Avoiding risky behaviors, such as injecting drugs and engaging in unprotected sex, can help prevent the transmission of viral infections.

Eating a healthy diet: Eating a healthy diet that is rich in fruits, vegetables, and other nutrients can help boost the immune system and reduce the risk of viral infections.

In conclusion, viral infections are infections that are caused by viruses, which are tiny infectious particles that can reproduce only inside the living cells of an organism. Antiviral medications, which are specific to each type of virus, are used to treat viral infections. There are several ways to reduce the risk of viral infections, including getting vaccinated, practicing good hygiene, avoiding risky behaviors, and eating a healthy diet. If you suspect that you have a viral infection, it is important to see a healthcare provider for proper diagnosis and treatment.

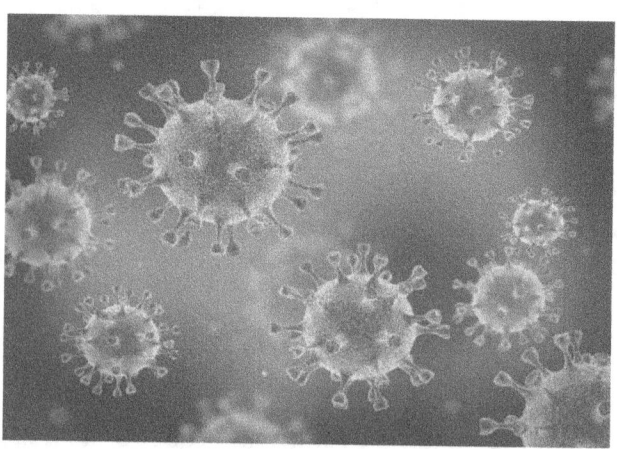

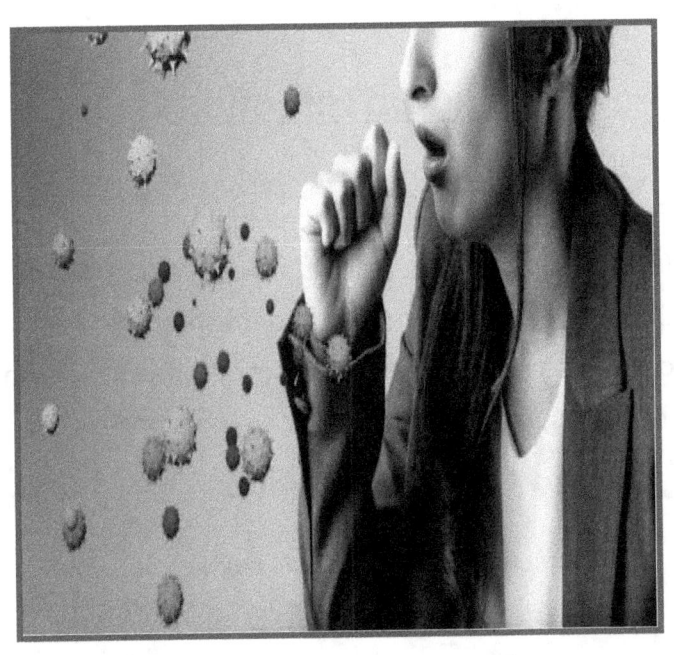

CHAPTER 9

Fungal Infections

Fungal infections are infections that are caused by fungi, which are a diverse group of microorganisms that include yeasts, molds, and mushrooms. Fungi can cause a wide range of infections, including skin infections, respiratory infections, and systemic infections.

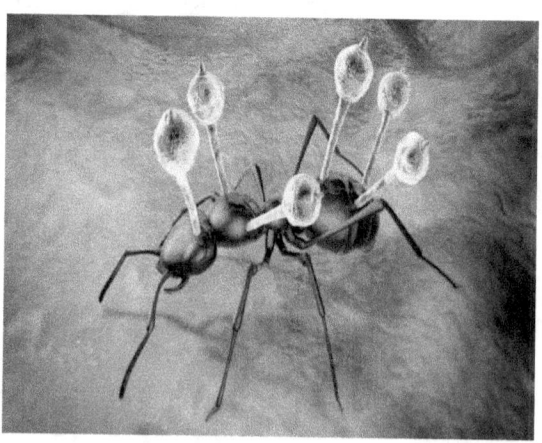

Some common types of fungal infections include:

Athlete's foot: Athlete's foot is a fungal infection of the skin on the feet that is characterized by red, itchy, and cracked skin. It is caused by a fungus called Trichophyton and is transmitted through contact with infected surfaces or with infected people. Athlete's foot can be treated with antifungal medications, such as terbinafine, and it can be prevented by avoiding contact with infected surfaces and by wearing shoes in public places.

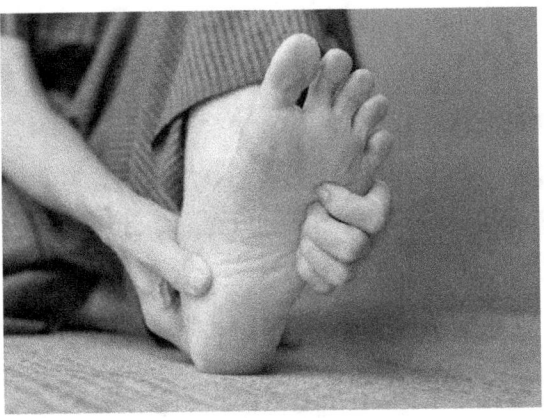

Ringworm: Ringworm is a fungal infection of the skin that is characterized by red, circular, and scaly patches on the skin. It is caused by a fungus called Dermatophytes and is transmitted through contact with infected people or with infected animals.

Ringworm can be treated with antifungal medications, such as terbinafine, and it can be prevented by avoiding contact with infected people and animals and by washing bedding and clothing in hot water.

Candidiasis: Candidiasis is a fungal infection that is caused by a yeast called Candida. It can affect various parts of the body, including the mouth, skin, and genital area, and it is characterized by symptoms such as itching, burning, and discharge. Candidiasis can be treated with antifungal medications, such as fluconazole, and it can be prevented by practicing good hygiene and by avoiding the use of tight-fitting clothing.

Fungal infections can be more challenging to treat than bacterial infections because fungi are more resistant to medications and can be more difficult to eliminate. They can also recur if the underlying cause, such as a weakened immune system, is not addressed.

In conclusion, fungal infections are infections that are caused by fungi, which are a diverse group of microorganisms that include yeasts, molds, and mushrooms. Fungal infections can affect various parts of the body and can be caused by a variety of fungi. Some common types of fungal infections include athlete's foot, ringworm, and candidiasis. Fungal infections can be more challenging to treat than bacterial infections, and they can recur if the underlying cause is not addressed. If you suspect that you have a fungal infection, it is important to see a healthcare provider for proper diagnosis and treatment.

Other types of fungal infections include:

Aspergillosis: Aspergillosis is a fungal infection that is caused by a mold called Aspergillus. It can affect various parts of the body, including the respiratory system, skin, and nails, and it is characterized by symptoms such as fever, cough, and shortness of breath. Aspergillosis can be treated with antifungal medications, such as voriconazole, and it can be prevented by avoiding contact with moldy or contaminated materials.

Pneumocystis pneumonia: Pneumocystis pneumonia is a fungal infection of the respiratory system that is caused by a fungus called Pneumocystis jirovecii. It is more common in people with weakened immune systems, such as people with HIV/AIDS, and it is characterized by symptoms such as fever, cough, and difficulty breathing. Pneumocystis pneumonia can be treated with antifungal medications, such as pentamidine, and it can be prevented with prophylactic medications in people with weakened immune systems.

Cryptococcosis: Cryptococcosis is a fungal infection that is caused by a yeast called Cryptococcus. It can affect various parts of the body, including the respiratory system and the central nervous system, and it is characterized by symptoms such as headache, fever, and confusion. Cryptococcosis can be treated with antifungal medications, such as amphotericin B, and it can be prevented by avoiding contact with contaminated materials.

In summary, fungal infections are infections that are caused by fungi, which are a diverse group of microorganisms that include yeasts, molds, and mushrooms. Fungal infections can affect various parts of the body and can be caused by a variety of fungi. Some common types of fungal infections include athlete's foot, ringworm, and candidiasis, while other types of fungal infections include aspergillosis, pneumocystis pneumonia, and cryptococcosis. Fungal infections can be more challenging to treat than bacterial infections, and they can recur if the underlying cause is not addressed. If you suspect that you have a fungal infection, it is important to see a healthcare provider for proper diagnosis and treatment.

In addition to the common fungal infections listed above, there are many other types of fungal infections that can affect people. Some of these infections are caused by fungi that are present in the environment, while others are caused by fungi that are normally present on the body but can cause infections when the body's defenses are weakened.

Some examples of other fungal infections include:

Blastomycosis: Blastomycosis is a fungal infection that is caused by a fungus called Blastomyces dermatitidis. It can affect various parts of the body, including the respiratory system, skin, and bones, and it is characterized by symptoms such as fever, cough, and weight loss. Blastomycosis can be treated with antifungal medications, such as itraconazole, and it can be prevented by avoiding contact with contaminated soil and water.

Histoplasmosis: Histoplasmosis is a fungal infection that is caused by a fungus called Histoplasma capsulatum. It can affect various parts of the body, including the respiratory system and the gastrointestinal tract, and it is characterized by symptoms such as fever, cough, and abdominal pain. Histoplasmosis can be treated with antifungal medications, such as itraconazole, and it can be prevented by avoiding contact with contaminated soil and bird droppings.

Sporotrichosis: Sporotrichosis is a fungal infection that is caused by a fungus called Sporothrix schenckii. It can affect the skin and the lymphatic system, and it is characterized by symptoms such as red, raised bumps on the skin and swelling of the lymph nodes. Sporotrichosis can be treated with antifungal medications, such as itraconazole, and it can be prevented by avoiding contact with contaminated soil and plants.

In summary, there are many types of fungal infections that can affect people, in addition to the common fungal infections such as athlete's foot, ringworm, and candidiasis.

CHAPTER 10

Prevention and Control of Infectious Diseases

Infectious diseases are diseases that are caused by pathogens, such as bacteria, viruses, and fungi, and that can be transmitted from one person to another or from animals to humans. Infectious diseases can have serious consequences, including death, and they can have a significant impact on public health and the economy. Therefore, preventing and controlling infectious diseases is important for the health and well-being of individuals and society.

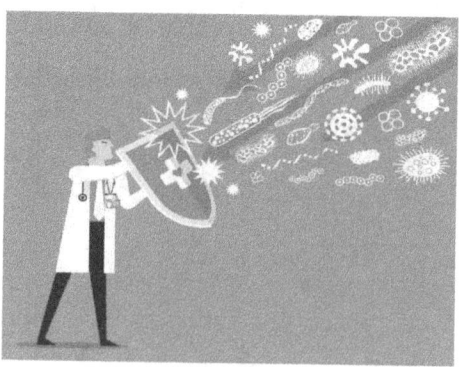

There are several ways to prevent and control infectious diseases, including:

Immunization: Immunization, or vaccination, is the process of administering a vaccine, which is a preparation of a pathogen or a part of a pathogen that is used to stimulate the immune system to produce antibodies that protect against the pathogen. Immunization can be used to prevent a wide range of infectious diseases, including measles, polio, and influenza.

Hygiene: Good hygiene practices, such as handwashing, can help prevent the transmission of infectious diseases. It is important to wash your hands frequently, especially before eating, after using the bathroom, and after coming into contact with infected people or objects.

Isolation: Isolation is the separation of infected people from non-infected people to prevent the spread of an infectious disease. Isolation can be used to prevent the transmission of highly contagious diseases, such as measles and tuberculosis.

Antimicrobial drugs: Antimicrobial drugs, such as antibiotics, antiviral medications, and antifungal medications, can be used to treat infectious diseases and to prevent the spread of infections.

Surveillance: Surveillance is the monitoring of infectious diseases to detect outbreaks and to track their spread. Surveillance can be used to identify trends in the incidence and prevalence of infectious diseases and to inform public health interventions.

In conclusion, preventing and controlling infectious diseases is important for the health and well-being of individuals and society. There are several ways to prevent and control infectious diseases, including immunization, hygiene, isolation, antimicrobial drugs, and surveillance. If you suspect that you have an infectious disease, it is important to see a healthcare provider for proper diagnosis and treatment.

Other measures that can be taken to prevent and control infectious diseases include:

Environmental interventions: Environmental interventions, such as improving sanitation and water quality, can help reduce the transmission of infectious diseases.

Personal protective measures: Personal protective measures, such as wearing masks and gloves, can help protect against the transmission of infectious diseases.

Quarantine: Quarantine is the separation and restriction of movement of people who have been exposed to an infectious disease to prevent the spread of the disease. Quarantine can be used to prevent the transmission of infectious diseases that have a long incubation period, such as Ebola.

Travel restrictions: Travel restrictions, such as border closures and travel bans, can be used to prevent the spread of infectious diseases.

Health education: Health education, such as providing information about the causes, symptoms, and prevention of infectious diseases, can help people understand how to protect themselves and others from infections.

In summary, there are several measures that can be taken to prevent and control infectious diseases, in addition to immunization, hygiene, isolation, antimicrobial drugs, and surveillance. These measures include environmental interventions, personal protective measures, quarantine, travel restrictions, and health education. It is important to follow recommended prevention and control measures to protect against infectious diseases and to reduce the spread of infections.

In addition to the prevention and control measures listed above, there are several strategies that can be used to reduce the impact of infectious diseases on individuals and communities. These strategies include:

Early detection: Early detection of infectious diseases can help initiate prompt treatment and prevent the spread of infections.

Outbreak response: An outbreak response is a coordinated effort to control and prevent the spread of an infectious disease. An outbreak response can include measures such as isolation, quarantine, and contact tracing.

Surveillance: Surveillance can help identify outbreaks of infectious diseases and track their spread. It can also be used to monitor the effectiveness of prevention and control measures.

Research: Research on infectious diseases can help identify the causes of infections, develop new treatments and vaccines, and improve our understanding of how infections spread and how they can be prevented.

Prevention and control programs: Prevention and control programs, such as immunization programs and hygiene education programs, can help reduce the incidence of infectious diseases and protect the health of individuals and communities.

In conclusion, there are several strategies that can be used to reduce the impact of infectious diseases on individuals and communities. These strategies include early detection, outbreak response, surveillance, research, and prevention and control programs. It is important to implement these strategies to protect against infectious diseases and to reduce their impact on individuals and communities.

In addition to the strategies mentioned above, there are several other factors that can affect the prevention and control of infectious diseases. These factors include:

The virulence of the pathogen: The virulence of the pathogen is a measure of its ability to cause disease. Pathogens with high virulence are more likely to cause severe disease and are more difficult to control.

The mode of transmission: The mode of transmission is the way in which a pathogen is transmitted from one person to another or from animals to humans. Understanding the mode of transmission of a pathogen can help identify the most effective prevention and control measures.

The susceptibility of the host: The susceptibility of the host is a measure of the likelihood that a person will become infected with a pathogen. Factors that can affect susceptibility include age, underlying health conditions, and immune status.

The availability of vaccines and treatments: The availability of vaccines and treatments can affect the prevention and control of infectious diseases. For example, if a vaccine or treatment is not widely available, it may be more difficult to control an infectious disease.

The social and economic factors: Social and economic factors, such as poverty, overcrowding, and inadequate access to healthcare, can affect the prevention and control of infectious diseases.

In conclusion, there are several factors that can affect the prevention and control of infectious diseases. These factors include the virulence of the pathogen, the mode of transmission, the susceptibility of the host, the availability of vaccines and treatments, and social and economic factors. Understanding these factors can help identify the most effective prevention and control measures.

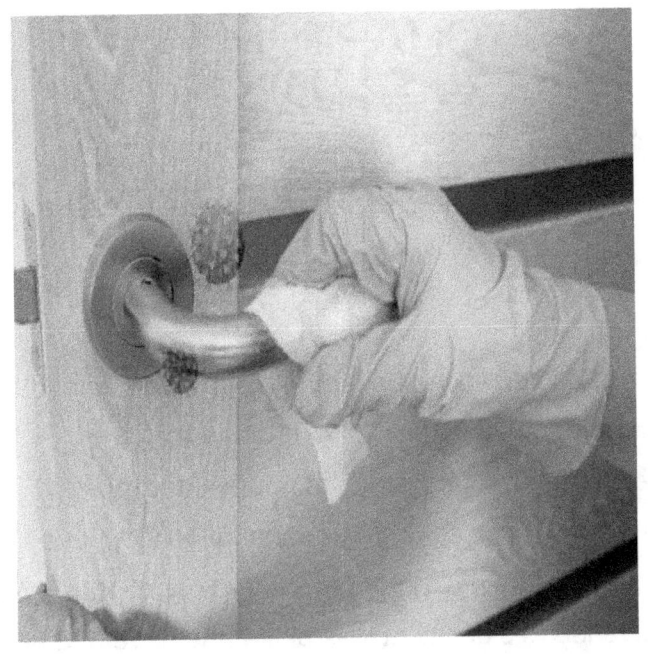

CHAPTER 11

The History of Infectious Diseases

Infectious diseases have had a significant impact on human history and have shaped the development of civilizations. Many infectious diseases, such as smallpox and influenza, have caused widespread epidemics and pandemics that have led to significant loss of life and have had a major impact on society.

Here are some examples of the history of infectious diseases:

Smallpox: Smallpox is an infectious disease caused by the variola virus that is characterized by fever, rash, and pustules on the skin. Smallpox has caused several epidemics and pandemics throughout history, including the devastating Third Pandemic in the late 19th and early 20th centuries, which is estimated to have killed 300 million people worldwide. Smallpox was declared eradicated in 1980 after a successful vaccination campaign.

Influenza: Influenza, or the flu, is an infectious disease caused by the influenza virus that is characterized by fever, cough, and muscle aches. Influenza has caused several pandemics throughout history, including the Spanish flu pandemic in 1918-1919, which is estimated to have killed 50 million people worldwide. Influenza continues to cause outbreaks and epidemics, and it can be prevented with vaccination.

Plague: Plague is an infectious disease caused by the bacterium Yersinia pestis that is characterized by fever, chills, and swollen lymph nodes. Plague has caused several epidemics and pandemics throughout history, including the Black Death in the 14th century, which is estimated to have killed 75-200 million people, or up to 50% of the population of Europe. Plague can be treated with antibiotics and can be prevented with measures such as avoiding contact with infected animals and people.

In conclusion, infectious diseases have had a significant impact on human history and have shaped the development of civilizations. Examples of infectious diseases that have caused epidemics and pandemics include smallpox, influenza, and plague. Understanding the history of infectious diseases can help inform current efforts to prevent and control these diseases.

Other examples of infectious diseases with a significant impact on human history include:

Tuberculosis: Tuberculosis is an infectious disease caused by the bacterium Mycobacterium tuberculosis that is characterized by fever, cough, and weight loss. Tuberculosis has affected humans for thousands of years and has been responsible for significant morbidity and mortality throughout history. Tuberculosis can be treated with antibiotics and can be prevented with measures such as vaccination and good hygiene practices.

Cholera: Cholera is an infectious disease caused by the bacterium Vibrio cholerae that is characterized by severe diarrhea, dehydration, and electrolyte imbalance. Cholera has caused several epidemics and pandemics throughout history, including the Seventh Cholera Pandemic in the 19th and 20th centuries, which is estimated to have killed millions of people worldwide. Cholera can be treated with oral rehydration therapy and antibiotics and can be prevented with measures such as improving water and sanitation.

HIV/AIDS: HIV/AIDS is an infectious disease caused by the human immunodeficiency virus (HIV) that is characterized by the progressive loss of immune function. HIV/AIDS has caused a global pandemic and has had a significant impact on public health and society. HIV/AIDS can be treated with antiretroviral therapy and can be prevented with measures such as safe sex practices and the use of condoms.

In summary, infectious diseases such as tuberculosis, cholera, and HIV/AIDS have had a significant impact on human history and have caused epidemics and pandemics. Understanding the history of these infectious diseases can help inform current efforts to prevent and control these diseases.

Other examples of infectious diseases with a significant impact on human history include:

Malaria: Malaria is an infectious disease caused by the parasite Plasmodium that is transmitted to humans through the bites of infected mosquitoes. Malaria has affected humans for thousands of years and has been responsible for significant morbidity and mortality throughout history. Malaria can be treated with antimalarial medications and can be prevented with measures such as the use of insect repellents and mosquito nets.

Yellow fever: Yellow fever is an infectious disease caused by the yellow fever virus that is transmitted to humans through the bites of infected mosquitoes. Yellow fever has caused several epidemics and pandemics throughout history, including the 1793 yellow fever epidemic in Philadelphia, which is estimated to have killed more than 5,000 people. Yellow fever can be prevented with vaccination and can be controlled with measures such as mosquito control.

Syphilis: Syphilis is an infectious disease caused by the bacterium Treponema pallidum that is transmitted through sexual contact, mother-to-child transmission, and direct contact with infected lesions. Syphilis has affected humans for centuries and has had a significant impact on public health and society. Syphilis can be treated with antibiotics and can be prevented with measures such as safe sex practices and the use of condoms.

In conclusion, infectious diseases such as malaria, yellow fever, and syphilis have had a significant impact on human history and have caused epidemics and pandemics. Understanding the history of these infectious diseases can help inform current efforts to prevent and control these diseases.

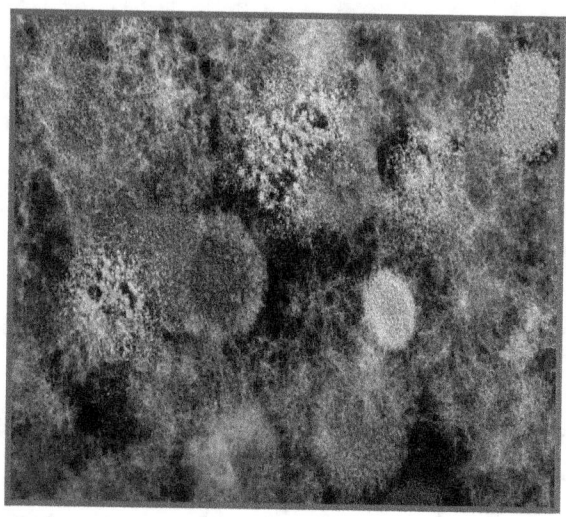

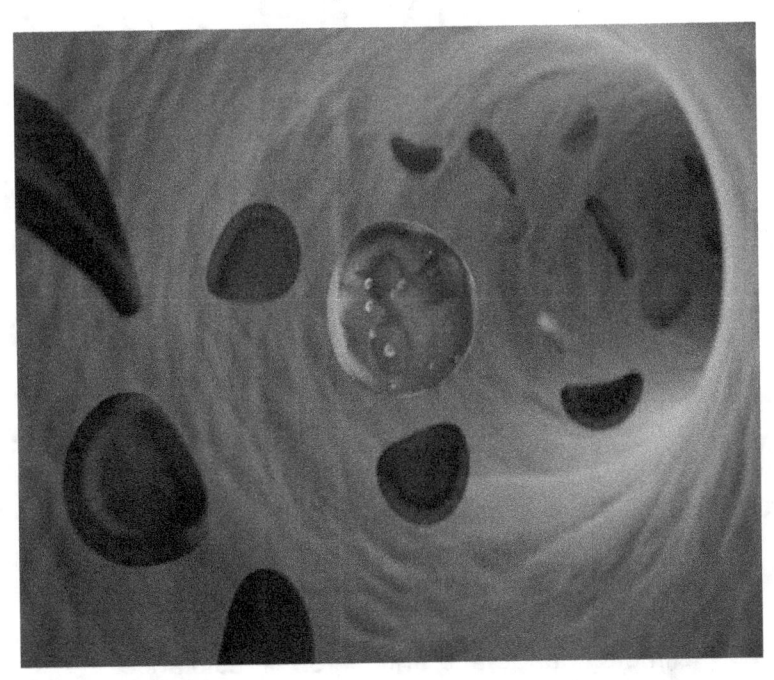

CHAPTER 12

The Future of Infectious Diseases

Infectious diseases will continue to be a major challenge for public health in the future. There are several factors that will shape the future of infectious diseases, including the emergence of new diseases, the evolution of existing diseases, and the impact of global health issues such as climate change and antimicrobial resistance.

Here are some examples of the future of infectious diseases:

Emergence of new diseases: The emergence of new diseases, such as SARS and Zika, has highlighted the need for ongoing surveillance and preparedness for new infectious threats. New diseases can emerge due to a variety of factors, such as the emergence of new pathogens, the spread of existing pathogens to new areas, and the evolution of existing pathogens.

Evolution of existing diseases: The evolution of existing diseases, such as influenza and HIV, can lead to the emergence of new strains of pathogens that are more virulent or more resistant to existing vaccines and treatments. This can pose a significant challenge for public health and can require the development of new vaccines and treatments.

Impact of climate change: Climate change can affect the transmission of infectious diseases, as changes in temperature and precipitation can impact the distribution of vectors, such as mosquitoes, and the survival of pathogens. This can lead to the emergence of new infectious diseases and the expansion of existing diseases to new areas.

Impact of antimicrobial resistance: Antimicrobial resistance is the ability of pathogens to survive exposure to antimicrobial drugs, such as antibiotics, and can lead to the emergence of drug-resistant infections. Antimicrobial resistance is a growing global threat and can have a significant impact on the ability to treat infectious diseases in the future.

In conclusion, the future of infectious diseases will be shaped by the emergence of new diseases, the evolution of existing diseases, the impact of climate change, and the impact of antimicrobial resistance. It is important to be prepared for new infectious threats and to address global health issues such as climate change and antimicrobial resistance in order to protect against infectious diseases in the future.

Other factors that may shape the future of infectious diseases include:

Increasing international travel and trade: Increasing international travel and trade can facilitate the spread of infectious diseases to new areas. This can pose a significant challenge for public health and can require the implementation of measures such as quarantine and travel restrictions to prevent the spread of infections.

Urbanization and population growth: Urbanization and population growth can lead to overcrowding and poor living conditions, which can increase the transmission of infectious diseases. This can be particularly challenging in low-income countries where access to healthcare and other resources may be limited.

Globalization of the food supply: The globalization of the food supply can increase the risk of the spread of foodborne illnesses, as food is often transported over long distances and may be produced in countries with less stringent food safety regulations.

Breakdown of healthcare systems: The breakdown of healthcare systems, such as during times of conflict or natural disasters, can increase the risk of the spread of infectious diseases. This can be particularly challenging in low-income countries where healthcare systems may be fragile and access to healthcare may be limited.

In summary, there are several factors that may shape the future of infectious diseases, including the emergence of new diseases, the evolution of existing diseases, the impact of climate change, the impact of antimicrobial resistance, increasing international travel and trade, urbanization and population growth, the globalization of the food supply, and the breakdown of healthcare systems. It is important to be prepared for these challenges and to implement measures to protect against infectious diseases in the future.

Other factors that may shape the future of infectious diseases include:

The impact of emerging technologies: Emerging technologies, such as genomics and synthetic biology, may have a significant impact on the future of infectious diseases. For example, genomics can be used to identify new pathogens and to understand how they evolve, which can inform the development of vaccines and treatments. Synthetic biology can be used to create new pathogens or to modify existing pathogens, which may have implications for bioterrorism and the spread of infections.

The impact of political and social factors: Political and social factors, such as conflicts, social unrest, and inequality, can have a significant impact on the transmission of infectious diseases. For example, conflicts and social unrest can disrupt healthcare systems and increase the risk of the spread of infections, while inequality can affect access to healthcare and other resources, which can impact the prevention and control of infectious diseases.

The impact of global economic factors: Global economic factors, such as trade and economic development, can have an impact on the transmission of infectious diseases. For example, economic development can lead to improvements in healthcare and other infrastructure, which can reduce the transmission of infections, while trade can facilitate the spread of infections to new areas.

In conclusion, there are several factors that may shape the future of infectious diseases, including the impact of emerging technologies, the impact of political and social factors, and the impact of global economic factors. It is important to consider these factors and to implement measures to protect against infectious diseases in the future.

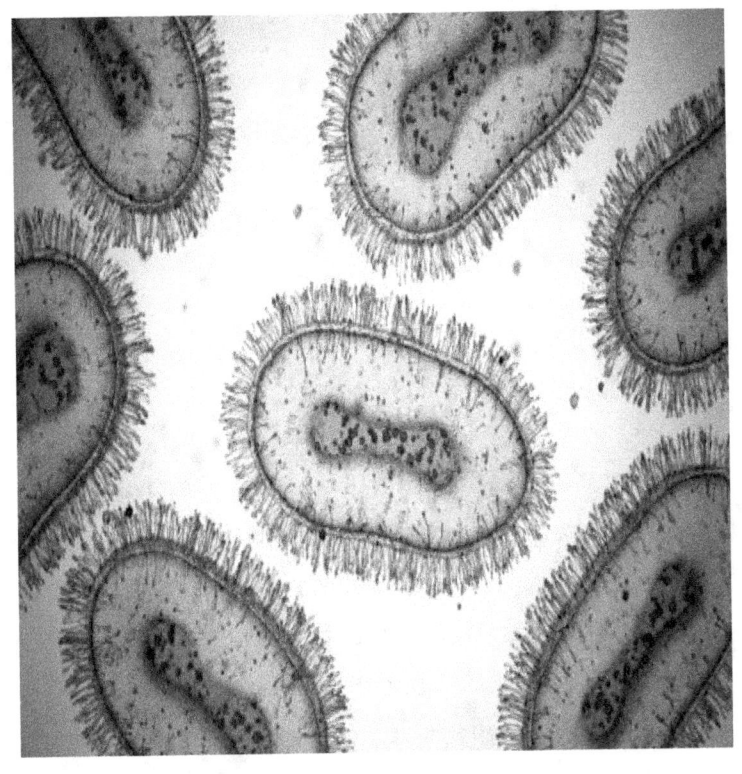

CHAPTER 13

Key Takeaways and Recommendations for the Public

Public Health Measures to Control Bacterial Infections:

Vaccination: Vaccination is a highly effective way to prevent bacterial infections. Vaccines work by stimulating the body's immune system to produce antibodies against a particular pathogen. This can help protect against bacterial infections such as pneumococcal disease, meningococcal disease, and Haemophilus influenzae type b (Hib).

Antibiotic use: Antibiotics can be used to treat bacterial infections and to prevent the spread of infections. However, the overuse and misuse of antibiotics can lead to the emergence of antibiotic-resistant bacteria, which can make infections more difficult to treat. It is important to use antibiotics responsibly and to follow the guidelines for their use.

Infection control: Infection control measures can help to reduce the transmission of bacterial infections. This can include measures such as hand hygiene, the use of personal protective equipment, and the isolation of infected individuals.

Surveillance: Surveillance systems can help to track the prevalence and spread of bacterial infections and to identify outbreaks. This can help public health authorities to implement appropriate control measures and to monitor the effectiveness of these measures.

Research: Research can help to identify new bacterial pathogens and to develop vaccines, treatments, and other prevention and control measures. This can help to improve our understanding of bacterial infections and to identify new strategies for their prevention and control.

Water and sanitation: Access to clean water and adequate sanitation can help to reduce the transmission of bacterial infections. This can include measures such as water treatment, sewage disposal, and the provision of toilets and handwashing facilities.

Food safety: Food safety measures can help to prevent the transmission of bacterial infections through the food supply. This can include measures such as proper food handling, cooking, and storage, as well as the regulation of food production and processing facilities.

Environmental factors: Environmental factors, such as overcrowding and poor living conditions, can increase the risk of bacterial infections. Public health measures such as improved housing, ventilation, and sanitation can help to reduce the transmission of infections.

Public health education: Public health education can help to inform individuals and communities about the risks and prevention of bacterial infections. This can include information on vaccination, hygiene practices, and other measures that can help reduce the transmission of infections.

In conclusion, there are several public health measures that can be used to control bacterial infections, including vaccination, antibiotic use, infection control, surveillance, research, water and sanitation, food safety, environmental factors, and public health education. These measures can help to reduce the transmission of infections and to protect individuals and communities from the negative impacts of bacterial infections.

Key Takeaways:

Infectious diseases continue to be a major challenge for public health and can have significant impacts on individuals, communities, and society.

There are several strategies that can be used to reduce the impact of infectious diseases, including early detection, outbreak response, surveillance, research, and prevention and control programs.

Factors that can affect the prevention and control of infectious diseases include the virulence of the pathogen, the mode of transmission, the susceptibility of the host, the availability of vaccines and treatments, and social and economic factors.

The future of infectious diseases will be shaped by the emergence of new diseases, the evolution of existing diseases, the impact of climate change, the impact of antimicrobial resistance, and other factors such as increasing international travel and trade, urbanization and population growth, the globalization of the food supply, and the breakdown of healthcare systems.

Recommendations for the Public:

Get vaccinated: Vaccination is a highly effective way to prevent infectious diseases. Talk to your healthcare provider about which vaccines are recommended for you and your family.

Practice good hygiene: Good hygiene practices, such as handwashing, can help to reduce the transmission of infectious diseases.

Stay informed: Stay informed about infectious diseases and the risks and prevention measures that are recommended. This can help you to protect yourself and your family from infections.

Seek medical attention if you are feeling unwell: If you are experiencing symptoms of an infectious disease, seek medical attention as soon as possible. Early diagnosis and treatment can help to reduce the severity and complications of an infection.

Support public health efforts: Support public health efforts to prevent and control infectious diseases, such as funding for research, vaccination programs, and other prevention and control measures.

CONCLUSION

Bacterial infections continue to be a major challenge for public health and can have significant impacts on individuals, communities, and society. These infections can range from mild to severe and can be caused by a variety of bacterial pathogens, such as Salmonella, E. coli, and Streptococcus.

There are several strategies that can be used to reduce the impact of bacterial infections, including vaccination, antibiotic use, infection control, surveillance, research, and public health measures such as water and sanitation, food safety, and environmental factors. These measures can help to prevent the transmission of infections and to protect individuals and communities from the negative impacts of bacterial infections.

However, the future of bacterial infections is uncertain and will be shaped by a variety of factors, including the emergence of new diseases, the evolution of existing diseases, the impact of climate change, and the impact of antimicrobial resistance. It is important to be prepared for these challenges and to implement measures to protect against bacterial infections in the future.

In conclusion, bacterial infections remain a significant challenge for public health and will continue to be a major focus of research and prevention efforts. By understanding the risks and prevention measures, and supporting public health efforts, individuals and communities can help to reduce the impact of bacterial infections and protect against these infections in the future.

www.ingramcontent.com/pod-product-compliance
Lightning Source LLC
Chambersburg PA
CBHW070240220526
45465CB00004B/1461